A Quick and Easy Guide on Dance

Mary Stephens

Published by ECONO Publishing Company, 2021.

While every precaution has been taken in the preparation of this book, the publisher assumes no responsibility for errors or omissions, or for damages resulting from the use of the information contained herein.

A QUICK AND EASY GUIDE ON DANCE

First edition. May 10, 2021.

Copyright © 2021 Mary Stephens.

ISBN: 979-8201787547

Written by Mary Stephens.

4 Great Ways to Learn to Dance

Moving is something that numerous individuals appreciate as a sporting pursuit as well as a fundamental piece of their wellness schedule. Dance is an extraordinary method to keep your body fit as a fiddle without feeling like you are by one way or another being rebuffed for getting a charge out of that additional scoop of frozen yogurt on your cone. Simultaneously, dance is likewise something that numerous individuals just find agreeable. Similarly as with most things throughout everyday life however, there are frequently good and bad manners by which you can make most dance moves and some of them probably won't be as useful for you as they might suspect. Consequently you truly need to look for qualified directions. Underneath you will discover four distinct techniques in which you can get the guidance you need to move your heart out.

Private Dance Instruction

Assuming you are in a monetary circumstance that takes into consideration this, this is the ideal alternative. With private exercises you will have one on one guidance and the immediate consideration of the educator. Private exercises give indisputably the most bang to your buck and will give the most quick result for your endeavors as you will move at your own speed and won't need to look out for different understudies to get up to speed or feel abandoned by understudies who have a higher starting degree of expertise.

Private exercises likewise give the chance to address explicit requirements and pain points with regards to your moving. This implies you will gain the correct route all along, furnished you went with a trustworthy educator who is truly learned. The advantages of private guidance are truly astounding when contrasted with a portion of the other accessible techniques for figuring out how to move.

Formal Group Dance Lessons

You can pursue bunch dance exercises at practically any age. There are not very many necessities and classes are offered for some, extraordinary experience levels too. In the event that you are an absolute fledgling there will be classes that will show you the rudiments and kick you off on your way. There are additionally classes that are intended to show progressed understudies more troublesome footwork and methods. A few group flourish in such classes on the grounds that there is some level of seriousness included. Agreeable rivalry is regularly an incredible helper for progress. Others notwithstanding, feel to some degree abandoned or unchallenged in such classes and would improve an alternate type of guidance.

Casual Group Dance Instruction

This is the kind of guidance you will frequently discover preceding moves in neighborhood ballrooms and dance club. The air is casual and the objective is to give an essential groundwork. Such a guidance will get ready to you to execute a couple of extremely essential moves and almost no else. This is mainstream in territories where line moving is normal to show benefactors how the moves engaged with explicit moves. This sort of guidance isn't suggested for the individuals who need a genuine measure of guidance with regards to move yet for the individuals who have a temporary premium and just need to gain proficiency two or three moves for no particular reason on a night out, this is ideal.

Video Dance Instruction

In all honesty, many would be artists are frozen at the actual considered somebody looking as they endeavor to get familiar with the moves needed for the moves they wish to execute. We live in a universe of sticklers be that as it may and assuming you end up being a fussbudget, video dance exercises might be the ideal wagered for your necessities and wishes. You will track down a wide choice of these video exercises on the web on the off chance that you will look. You will even discover numerous that are intended to instruct dance for the sole motivation behind wellness while others show dance for the sole reason for the sake of entertainment.

The heading you take with regards to figuring out how to move is totally dependent upon you. The a wide range of kinds of classes offer appeal to the various sorts of individuals on the planet today. In the event that one sort of class worked for everybody wishing to take classes, there would be no requirement for the various kinds of dance classes. Truly not every person learns best in a similar circumstance. Select the learning technique that you feel will be best for you and begin figuring out how to move today.

7 Great Reasons to Dance

With regards to move there are a lot of brilliant reasons that individuals choose for dance. The reality stays that very not many of us figure out how to join dance into our lives almost however much we ought to. There are numerous superb motivations to move and they don't all need abundant measures of liquor and somebody with a camcorder ready for America's Funniest Home Videos significance.

Underneath I will propose 7 extraordinary motivations to fuse dance into your life as regularly as could be expected. I trust that you will acknowledge a portion of these and track down a couple of reasons of your own to move all the more regularly.

Love

There are not many more prominent motivations to move than to show your affection for your accomplice. You don't need to restrict your moving to your wedding night or an evening out with companions. All you need to hit the dance floor with the one you love is some acceptable music and a tad of floor space. Dance while you plan supper, wash dishes, or in light of the fact that it's pouring outside. Yet, hit the dance floor with the one you cherish and do it regularly to keep those blazes consuming.

Bliss

We generally hear individuals looking at moving for euphoria yet how frequently do we truly witness that? What a disgrace it is that we really accept scarcely any open doors to move in our general public. Moving is an overt gesture of happiness that is quite often irresistible. Offer your bliss with the world and you very well could discover they will move alongside you. Regardless of whether they don't, you ought to in any event be secure in the way that as of now in time you are a lot more joyful than they are.

Fun

When is the last time you've moved? Was it fun? I have discovered not very many individuals (well other than young men) who didn't have a good time while moving. The reality of the situation is that moving is enjoyable. Regardless of whether you are line moving or attempting the Tango it is extraordinary enjoyable to move.

Being a tease

What an awesome method to be a tease moving can be! In the event that you haven't attempted it with the one you love, there is no better time than right now to do as such. Track down some incredible fun and coquettish music and dance for the one you love. In case you're truly fortunate, you may even persuade them to participate.

To Make Your Children Laugh

Truly, there could be no greater explanation on the earth than this to move. My children love to see me dance the moves that were well known back when dinosaurs meandered the earth and offer their more current moves with me. It's an extraordinary method to make the most of your youngsters before they choose your malevolence or during those uncommon minutes when you might be nearly impartial in their feelings.

Wellness

While moving does a ton to ease up the temperament and raise your spirits it can likewise help your heart in alternate manners also. Moving is an extraordinary method to get up and moving that doesn't feel like it is truly work out. This implies that you can help your heart by moving a short time each day. The more you dance, the better you will feel and the better your heart will turn into.

Meet New People

In the event that you choose to take exercises for moving, you will find that you can meet a lot of extraordinary new individuals. Moving is an incredible way that numerous individuals are finding to have a great time and stay fit. This implies that an ever increasing number of individuals are joining nearby dance classes for these very reasons. You may build up some deep rooted companionships through your dance exercises that you would have passed up something else.

Obviously there are a lot more reasons that various individuals take up dance. Truth be told, you may track down an all-together unique motivation to take up dance for yourself. Whatever your explanation you choose to move, do it regularly and have some good times all the while.

Ballet performance Classes for All Ages

For the individuals who are keen on dance classes, expressive dance exercises specifically, there are numerous choices from which to pick. In many zones you will discover expressive dance exercises that are accessible to understudies of any age just as a wide scope of involvement levels. Starting grown-ups are normal today as an ever increasing number of individuals find the wellness advantages of fusing dance, like artful dance into their wellness schedule.

For youngsters, ballet production exercises frequently start very early now and then as right on time as the age of three. There are no vertical cutoff points on artful dance exercises now apparently. However long the understudies are genuinely ready to do the moves and want to do as such, I sincerely can't see them being gotten some distance from a studio that is really devoted to sharing the energy of dance.

Ballet performance exercises can show significant exercises to individuals of any age that work out in a good way past your regular dance moves. Indeed, perhaps the best exercise that ballet production classes train understudies is the exercise of control. Control is needed to accomplish significance with regards to expressive dance or some other sort of dance or game. The previous we gain proficiency with this exercise the good we will be. I suggest getting your kids associated with a type of imaginative development dance or vaulting course as near the age of 3 as the dance schools in your space permits to ingrain the standards of training as ahead of schedule as could be expected.

Ballet performance classes for little ones is additionally a significant apparatus for assisting them with acquiring significant socialization abilities like sharing consideration, alternating, and functioning as a component of a gathering. Your youngster will anticipate the experience every single week and it will consume off a smidgen of their overabundance energy. As a parent I can't in any way, shape or form pressure the significance of this every so often as it would give the uncommon evening where there are no contentions when sleep time moves around.

As your youngster ages and advances in their artful dance schooling you will find that your kid is finding out increasingly more about the significance of support inside a gathering, the worth of control, and maybe in particular great confidence. These exercises are not to be trifled with. Another incredible thing about ballet performance classes for kids and adolescents is that it keeps them up and dynamic each exercise they take and consistently that they spend rehearsing is a second that they aren't lounging around thoughtlessly staring at the TV and playing computer games or stuffing lousy nourishment into their mouths.

For grown-ups, the worth of ballet performance exercises or some other type of dance besides is similar as the worth it has for youngsters and teenagers. Control is a significant expertise to master and cultivate at whatever stage in life. Indeed, even those with some level of control as of now can frequently utilize another support strategy and dance will build up sure order in an individual. Another tremendous advantage is to ballet performance exercises for grown-ups is the way that it is additionally keeping you dynamic and on your feet.

Ballet performance is a type of activity that ends up working many significant muscle bunches on the double. Expressive dance is an intriguing type of activity for some, who might somehow stay away from practice all together. The effortless stream and type of artful dance are likewise moves that power the artist to curve and stretch while keeping up brilliant stance. The exercise might be lower in sway than numerous different exercises anyway it is as yet consuming calories at a lot more noteworthy rate than lounging around the house staring at the TV. Ballet performance classes are an extraordinary action to seek after at practically any age gave you are in appropriate wellbeing to deal with the afflictions of ballet performance.

Formal Dancing is Making Waves

Up to this point, partner dancing regularly achieved mental pictures of old couples moving two creeps from their walkers. Be that as it may, lately, couples dancing has built up another, cooler, hotter picture and individuals of any age are standing up and focusing.

Films, for example, Strictly Ballroom and Shall We Dance have contributed incredibly to the more current kinder picture that formal dancing is creating in the United States. As a work of art, formal dance is an excellent incredible sight. Especially when watching those take an interest on a cutthroat level.

In light of the thorough preparing that is associated with serious formal dancing, numerous couples that partake frequently believe this to be a game in excess of a style of dance or way of imaginative articulation. The term DanceSport is frequently utilized regarding couples dancing in the International Style.

There are numerous styles of dance that fall under the flag of traditional dancing. A portion of these moves are frequently viewed as the most delightful to look just as among the most erotic styles of dance in the world. No one but you can choose for yourself if traditional dance is something that may intrigue you. I do, be that as it may, urge you to assess the different styles and topics before singularly choosing to preclude all partner dance as a potential interest.

Global Style

Under the International Style of partner dance there are two fundamental classes of dance. They are Standard and Latin. The Standard style is regularly hallmarked by Fred and Ginger kind of clothing. By this I imply that the style of dress is formal with men in covers with streaming tails and vests while the ladies wear exceptionally rich outfits as a feature of their ensembles. Latin dance is undeniably more sexy in music, disposition, and clothing. Men wear tight fitting pieces of clothing and ladies wear practically nothing.

Standard

Not exclusively is the style of dance among Standard and Latin altogether different yet in addition the styles of dance. In Standard partner dancing you will track down the accompanying moves: the Quickstep, the Slow Foxtrot, the Tango, the Viennese Waltz, and the Waltz. The Tango for some is the feature of the Standard occasion while others have a profound appreciation for the specialized characteristics of the numerous Standard moves of formal dancing.

Latin

For the more youthful age, the Latin bit of rivalries is the enthusiastically expected occasion. The style of dance is fascinating and passionate just as unbelievably excellent to watch. The state of mind this style of dance brings not exclusively to the artists yet in addition to the crowd is practically discernible. The fan top choices of Latin dance incorporate the Cha, Paso Doble, the Rumba, the Samba, and Jive dance. This type of dance is surely with regards to the possibility that dance is rapidly turning into a game. The energy needed for these moves is amazing similar to the wellness level needed to wear the outfits.

American Style

The American standard with regards to move is somewhat not the same as the International Style. The two classifications for American Style are Smooth and Rhythm. There are different contrasts also. In International Style the couples are needed to stay in a shut development. For American Style traditional dance these necessities are fairly loose to consider inventive utilization of footwork. The progression designs for Latin or Rhythm dance are likewise somewhat not quite the same as in the International Style of partner dancing however the exotic nature of the music, ensembles, and developments are a lot of something similar.

Smooth

The smooth segment of the American Style of partner dance incorporates the Foxtrot, the Tango, the Viennese Waltz, and the Waltz.

Cadence

In American Style Ballroom dance the Rhythm segment of the dance incorporates the accompanying: the Bolero, the Cha, East Coast Swing, the Mambo, and the Rumba. The crowd actually appreciates the force of Latin dance and Latin impact however there are different impacts too. These are as yet an eagerly awaited crowd top choice in many rivalries.

As should be obvious, formal dance has taken on another power as of late. In the event that you have assumptions of what formal dance truly is, it is time you saw with your own eyes how arousing this style of dance can truly be.

Hip twirl Basics

Oriental Dance, otherwise called hip twirling is one of, if not the most arousing styles of dance. It is likewise quite possibly the most helpful types of dance there is healthwise. Notwithstanding the incredible calorie consuming effect of hip twirling there are other medical advantages that this type of dance has gotten well known for throughout the long term.

Hip twirl has a long and pleased history tracing all the way back to the beginning of human progress. This style of dance has in its set of experiences been utilized as both a demonstration of love and a demonstration of enticement. Not generally in rejection of the either as this type of dance is accepted by certain religions to be a lift for fruitfulness of recently married couples.

Hip twirl is a style of dance that doesn't expect members to be in ideal state of being to start. Indeed, the low effect nature of this type of development settles on it a superb decision for the individuals who are not fit as a fiddle regardless. This type of dance works the muscles tenderly with the jostling impacts of effect high impact exercise and other exercise strategies. It likewise works the stomach, which is frequently the pain point for some, who aren't in the awesome shape. You ought to likewise find that you will reinforce your back through hip twirl as you progress. This will likewise assist with pretty much every part of your actual wellness schedule. All the more critically for the individuals who are a bit (or a ton) in a bad way is the hip twirl consumes a normal of 300 calories 60 minutes. This implies that in the event that you practice one hour daily you are consuming more than 2,000 calories each week.

For the individuals who praise their womanhood, there could be no more excellent type of dance to communicate that delight. Hip twirl has a long history as a festival of being female. From being utilized in functions in the sanctuary to being utilized to tempt and lure the accidental hip twirl is a festival of just being a young lady.

On the off chance that you are reluctant to start your hip twirl exercises in a class brimming with different people you can generally pick to buy recordings and DVD exercises. There are large numbers of these exercises from which to pick, even exercises that attention on the psychological and additionally recuperating parts of Oriental dance if that is the place where you believe you need to center your endeavors. Hip twirling is a lot of fun as well as being a fair type of getting genuinely necessary active work.

In the event that you intend to hip twirl, you ought to comprehend that the ensemble is important for what sets the mind-set or the tone. While you needn't bother with every one of the fancy odds and ends, the overall agreement is that exposing your midsection places you in the perspective that is generally appropriate for hip twirling. Hence it is suggested that you wear garments that exposed your tummy, for example, low-ascent yoga pants and a games bra or some other gut uncovering shirt for your training meetings. This likewise helps your teacher check whether you are taking the actions accurately.

On the off chance that you choose to participate in hip twirling classes, congrats! You will join a notable gathering of ladies that date back to what many accept is the absolute starting point of time. You ought to likewise have another pastime that is both engaging and solid.

Dance Revolution

The individuals who aren't enormous enthusiasts of gaming frameworks may not understand that Dance Revolution is really a computer game for the Playstation 2 gaming framework that really has overwhelmed the business. It was one of, if not the absolute first endeavors of the gaming business to battle the possibility that messing around denied offspring of the active work that is so critical to their general wellbeing and prosperity.

The arrangement was to present a game in which the players were scored dependent on their capacity to move as per the bearings of the game. On the off chance that you haven't attempted this game, let me be quick to disclose to you that it requires some extravagant footwork and more than some level of exclusive focus. The truly cool thing about this game is that you can change the degree of trouble and consolidate games with companions who have a similar game for an opposition. Rivalry with yourself is fine and dandy yet pulverizing your companions with your dance abilities is far and away superior.

This is a game that turns out to cross generational hindrances in any case and making a significant sprinkle in doing as such. Moms and fathers are contending with children and girls and the bets are very phenomenal. I realize I've been known to win possibly 14 days off from washing dishes as the consequence of an animating round of agreeable rivalry. The incongruity is that I'm not actually that great at the game. It is a lot of fun however and I feel less regretful about allowing the children to play this game for an hour than I do about permitting them to play some "all your base are have a place with us" kind of game for 60 minutes.

The wide ubiquity of the game ought to be totally clear in all the 'knock off' variants of this game that have effectively overwhelmed the market. I do hope to see more games along this line sooner rather than later especially with the new Nintendo Wii framework causing a ripple effect for the actual idea of large numbers of their games. The expectation is unquestionably that the Playstation Dance Revolution. We have effectively seen circle back to Dance Revolution 2, Dance Revolution Extreme, and Dance Revolution SuperNova. I can just foresee that Playstation will endeavor to carry this effective line to the debilitated Playstation 3 soon.

To the extent the exercise truth of this game goes you will find that it offers a superb vigorous exercise and extraordinary activities for your legs. The arms are truly dependent upon you generally. In the event that you decided to approach in a stream dance kind of technique your arms are probably going to get an incredible great level of an exercise that your legs will get. In any case on the off chance that you put everything into your dance moves, the unrest will be every one of the calories you consume just as the reinforcing and conditioning you oversee as a side advantage.

While not very many of us consider computer games to be an extraordinary wellspring of wellbeing or wellness, this game might be the one special case for the standard. Who might have at any point figured you could get these things thus substantially more from playing a computer game. Before you know it they'll come out with Mountain Dew that is a wellbeing drink.

Dance for Children

With regards to our youngsters, we need to give them the world. Numerous young ladies and some young men show an early interest in dance and you ought not stress over sexual orientation generalizations at youthful ages particularly. The advantages of dance for youngsters far exceed any potential generalizing that may occur as the outcome. Kids, regardless of whether male or female can take in numerous things from dance classes that go a long ways past reasonable applications in their moving. These life exercises are essential for the allure of dance classes to guardians all throughout the planet.

Dance Teaches Important Lessons

Similar as group activities, dance for kids can show some priceless and significant exercises. Order and restraint are vital character characteristics with regards to move. You should practice and you should stand firm on yourself in the legitimate footings for the moves you need to take. Your kid will likewise figure out how to alternate, to share consideration, and to help out others. These are vital abilities for a little youngster to create and move classes are frequently offered for kids at a lot more youthful age than many group activities. Your kid will likewise get familiar with the significance of being a piece of a gathering as numerous moves include everybody in the class.

Dance classes additionally show your kids music, cadence, and beat. Your kid will turn out to be more planned as the aftereffect of their dance classes and these classes are an extraordinary manner by which to empower actual wellness and exercise. By showing your youngster from the get-go in life the significance of development and wellness you will ingrain in that person the apparatuses the individual will require to remain in great shape throughout their life.

Dance for youngsters will likewise help assemble confidence in your kid as the individual achieves new objectives and assignments every week. You should observe intently in any case and ensure that this isn't misfiring by having your kid in a style of dance that the person in question finds baffling. While you do need your kid's dance classes to introduce a test you additionally don't need them to be such a large amount of a test that your kid isn't appreciating them by the same token.

You ought to likewise remember that on the off chance that you are thinking about a drawn out obligation to move classes and serious dance, the monetary responsibility could be huge. This is anything but a modest choice to group activities. Truth be told, a remarkable inverse is valid at more established and more aggressive degrees of dance. Not exclusively are the monetary responsibilities genuine yet in addition the responsibility of time. Dance is a brilliant strategy for showing your kid numerous significant abilities that will extraordinarily help build up the personality of your kid. That being said you ought to know that if this becomes something in which your kid is particularly capable, you may track down that the expenses are more than you had envisioned.

You will likewise find that there are a wide range of kinds of dance that are offered for kids. Among a portion of the more well known are artful dance, jazz, tap, ethnic moves, hip jump, and hip twirling just to give some examples. More youthful kids will presumably take a couple of imaginative development classes as opposed to bouncing into one explicit style. This allows your youngsters an opportunity to encounter various styles of dance and to find which moves are more charming and characteristic inclination to them.

With everything taken into account, dance for kids is an incredible method to construct priceless social abilities. Considerably more critically in any case, it is a chance to show your kids the significance of being important for an option that could be bigger than themselves. This is something extremely couple of youngsters truly comprehend and that will work well for them as they develop and become grown-ups. In the event that you are searching for an astounding studio that encourages dance for youngsters you should focus on those studios that place an accentuation on self-improvement for your kid more than serious freedoms, especially in more youthful years. As your kid's abilities and eagerness for dance develop you can generally decide to move your youngster to a more rivalry centered studio.

Dance for Fun

We as a whole have things in life we love to do. A portion of these things we love more than others. Moving is something that large numbers of us, as we age, neglect to make an opportunity to appreciate. In any case, moving is one of those straightforward joys in life that can likewise remind us to grin, to play, to twirl around until we get unsteady, and in particular to appreciate the straightforwardness of having some good times without the concern of work, family, or funds disrupting everything.

It costs almost no in many homes to just turn the radio on, draw the shades and dance. You can hit the dance floor with your loved one, your deep rooted accomplice, and surprisingly your kids. You don't need to stress over anybody watching and on the off chance that they are watching you should take feel sorry for that they are investing their energy agonizing over the thing you are doing instead of moving around and appreciating life to its fullest.

Local Americans had the correct thought with regards to moving. Leave the beat alone your guide and basically dance. They moved as a methods for love, to communicate accommodation to their divine beings, to lift up their divine beings, to show their delight, and as an overt gesture of sadness. They moved for adoration and they moved for war. Moving to them was however normal as strolling may be to a considerable lot of us and significant methods for articulating their thoughts as unique individuals as well as a component of a bigger and brought together gathering.

On the off chance that you have never moved for no particular reason, it's an ideal opportunity to look at the different styles of dance and see what offers to you as a style of dance. There are numerous kinds of dance and a wide range of styles of music for those different styles.

Line Dancing

Line moving is a way of moving in which artists line up and dance together by making a similar dance ventures simultaneously. It has cleared the country as well as is rapidly advancing all throughout the planet as a superb wellspring of moving fun. It's additionally an extraordinary method to mingle and meet new individuals. While line moving was essentially restricted to blue grass music at the outset it has immediately advanced into different styles of music also. Numerous bars, ballrooms, and clubs will offer line moving exercises on sluggish business evenings to support additional business. Line moving can be delighted in by the two people.

Square Dancing

This style of dance has a fairly long history and has encountered a decent level of advancement over the recent many years. While it was once held for cultivator downs and such square moving is rapidly turning into a side interest for some individuals across America and an incredible method to go through an evening and become more acquainted with other people who share this leisure activity. This way of moving is best delighted in by couples and can be such incredible fun in the event that you let your hair down a piece while taking an interest.

Hip twirling

Hip twirling can be appreciated by people however it is most normally connected with ladies. Except if you incorporate the appreciation that goes alone with observing as opposed to taking part and all things considered the men may really dwarf the ladies. Hip twirling is an exceptionally extraordinary and sexual type of dance that is quite often a crowd of people thrill ride. It might require a very long time to consummate your hip twirling moves and many examination this style of dance their whole lives however it is an incredible active work that is loads of fun.

Moving for entertainment only isn't unquestionably the best motivation to move by a long shot, yet it is excessively frequently not the explanation that individuals dance. Individuals dance for rivalry, for work out, and for some different reasons yet not almost regularly enough do we take the actions basically for the joy of doing as such. In the event that I could make one idea to everybody perusing it is this. Go out and dance for the sheer delight of moving.

Dance to Your Health

We as a world are more mindful than any other time of the significance of actual wellness to our general wellbeing. While we stay mindful of the requirement for active work very a considerable lot of us view far as too couple of motivations to join actual work into our day by day lives and schedules. There are numerous reasons that we delay in this specific exertion. For quite a while is the characterizing factor while others will promptly concede that they have no appreciation at all for those exercises that ring a bell when exercise is thought of.

Whatever your justification not joining exercise and actual work into your day by day schedule, have you thought about moving for your wellbeing? There are a wide range of awesome motivations to move however I can consider not very many that would be superior to moving for your wellbeing and actual prosperity. The uplifting news with regards to moving is that in many examples it doesn't feel like you are getting exercise and the consuming of calories doesn't sting close to as much when you're having a good time consuming them.

Moving has advanced an incredible arrangement and keeping in mind that the historical backdrop of dance is a long and honorable history. Indeed, one may add, a very masculine history for those men who haven't considered moving previously.

Advantages of Dancing

As well as consuming calories, something beneficial for health food nuts all over, moving additionally reinforces your muscles and bones. It can give either a low effect or high effect exercise as per your desires and the music you select, it very well may be engaging and feel like fun instead of a task—this implies you are bound to really do it than numerous other exercise projects, and it can help tone all spaces of your body as opposed to zeroing in on one specific territory as numerous activities do.

Moving additionally gives a magnificent chance to mingle and meet others in the event that you take classes while in the process assisting you with acquiring a superior feeling of equilibrium and beauty (those like me who have definitely no feeling of elegance could enormously profit by this by itself). Moving, and the active work alone can help you avert potential sicknesses that are regularly connected with overabundance weight and too minimal actual work. Indeed, even just thirty minutes of dance 4 days seven days can achieve significant outcomes with regards to your general wellbeing and prosperity.

More critically anyway than any of these advantages of moving referenced above moving is entertaining. This implies that you will appreciate life a bit, snicker a bit, and coincidentally work a little actual wellness into your existence without feeling like you are languishing over the purpose of doing as such. Such countless individuals get almost no actual work since they don't consider physical to be as fun.

On the off chance that you are thinking about what kind of dance is appropriate for you, there are numerous from which to pick. Square moving is incredible diversion for couples as are assembly hall and swing moving. Line moving, contra square moving, stopping up, and tap moving can be extraordinary fun in bigger gatherings or as a member in a class. In the event that you need something somewhat hotter for your dance endeavors you can generally attempt Salsa moving, Flamenco moving, or hip twirling.

On the off chance that you live in or around a generally enormous local area all things considered, you can discover classes or educators for private exercises for every one of these types of dance without any problem. You would like to ensure that anybody you take exercises from understands what they are doing. You can likewise glance in your neighborhood paper for square moving gatherings or bars or clubs that offer line moving classes on assigned evenings during the week.

Regardless of whether you have been moving for your entire life or are a position amateur with regards to moving, this is an incredible method to bring actual wellness into your life and improving your wellbeing without feeling like you are truly working for it or encountering a feeling of fear at the extremely thought.

Moving Through History

Through history we have seen numerous developments of dance. A portion of these old moves and ceremonies are as yet polished today by the individuals who honor their strict or social narratives while many have tragically been lost all through the ages. A certain something anyway stays steady. Dance has consistently assumed a significant part in the social orders, incredible and little, of the world.

Tracing all the way back to the start of written history moving has been a crucial piece of society. Dance was engaged with festivities and arrangements for war. Dance was essential for customs and services of love. Dance was essential for daily routine and we experience in a general public today that appears to progressively name dance as a type of amusement in excess of a lifestyle. Maybe that is important for the explanation we have a developing mindfulness with regards to discouragement in light of the fact that less individuals are encountering the delight of dance.

Did you realize that the Spartan heroes utilized dance in their arrangements for the fight to come? They consolidated a 'weapons dance' that was planned not exclusively to acquaint themselves with their weaponry yet additionally to assist them with being lithe when utilizing them. Trust me when I say that not many at any point tried inquiry the manliness of Spartans on the war zone. These troopers were ready for war and an enormous level of that is the aftereffect of their weapon moves as mental and actual groundwork for the specialty of taking up arms. With the Spartans war was undoubtedly a fine art.

Oriental Dance was regular during what has gotten known as Biblical occasions and remains today an exceptionally significant type

33

of dance. Indeed, Oriental Dances, additionally alluded to as Belly Dancing, is by all accounts encountering a resurrection of sorts as its ubiquity has spread all throughout the planet as of late. This style of dance has been utilized as a component of strict functions just as to allure sweethearts and affect desire and sometimes to address ripeness. Oriental Dance has a long and interesting history that is definitely worth further examination on the off chance that you are of the brain to do as such.

In Medieval occasions dance was a social necessity by those of means or holding status. Truth be told, what we know as partner dancing today started during this period and has advanced a little throughout the long term while maintaining its unique structure somewhat. The congregation at that point anyway disliked moving however numerous individuals from the congregation endured moving as well as taken an interest in these moves. After a lot of pressing factor from the general population the congregation did ultimately acknowledge and accept dance.

The developments for the archaic dance steps were supposed to be somewhat basic and dreary. While a portion of the moves of the day were performed by couples there were numerous processional or line moves that were mainstream during this period too. Who realized the line moving had a long and recognized history?

As times have developed so has dance. In the present society dance is regularly restricted to rivalries, celebrations, and gatherings instead of the conspicuousness it once held in the public arena. The uplifting news in this is that dance is no longer for some in the public eye an action that is exclusively saved for the most affluent among us. In spite of the fact that admittance to move exercises, classes, recordings, and so forth is in no way, shape or form strong confirmation that they will be used the reality stays that not very many urban communities in the United States don't offer dance classes that are at any rate barely reasonable for the individuals who partake. Cutthroat dance is another matter all together in any case and can bring a huge sticker price to the individuals who are uninformed or found napping. Sporting dance notwithstanding, frequently costs minimal more than the music needed with which to move and the will to move somewhere inside. We live in a country of chance, don't waste the chance we need to fuse the basic joy of moving into our day by day lives.

I Hope You Dance

There are numerous things in life we can do to show feelings and let others know how we feel. A few group sing, a few group compose verse and writing, some retreat inside themselves and hold everything inside. Others dance. Dance has for quite a long time been an approach to communicate a wide scope of feelings. It is a magnificent source for the feelings that on occasion our brains essentially can't measure. Moving is a technique where you can work through those feelings and somewhat proceed onward with your life notwithstanding enthusiastic disturbance.

In all honesty, numerous individuals accept that hip twirling (or Oriental Dance) brings passionate recuperating as well as actual mending for certain conditions. Dance is notable as a type of activity yet hip twirling is a kind of moving that is body cordial. This implies that you don't should be in the awesome actual shape to go into such a moving. You won't need to stress over weight on your joints because of high effect moves that different types of dance require. You ought to likewise take note of that the developments in oriental dance these moves are smooth and common.

Among the medical advantages you can insight through Oriental Dance are improved flow, lower pulse, improved joint wellbeing, and the consuming of calories. Some accept that notwithstanding the medical advantages referenced over that Oriental Dance can likewise help improve whiplash side effects and back issues. On the off chance that you are thinking about hip twirling to address such side effects you definitely should talk with your primary care physician prior to doing as such and ensure that you have an exceptionally qualified educator.

With regards to Oriental Dance, actual mending isn't the lone kind of recuperating that is regularly capable. Numerous artists additionally wind up relinquishing the pressure and strain in their lives just as some very horrible issues that have been in their past that may keep frequenting them long after. Thus, Oriental Dance is in some cases suggested for medicines of intense subject matters just as actual diseases.

There are vides, for example, Healing Dance that will permit you to become familiar with a portion of the fundamental moves at home. In any case, on the off chance that you include the assets inside your local area there is actually nothing that can supplant taking dance exercises with a gathering of ladies. You will track down that these ladies come in all shapes and estimates and from a wide range of monetary, physical, and profound foundations. It's a hardening experience to get together with different ladies for physical or potentially enthusiastic mending, for example, an Oriental Dance class will give.

Notwithstanding the Oriental mending dance there is additionally the African recuperating dance. This is somewhat more high effect in nature and spotlights on recuperating through articulations of bliss. This is a very inspiring type of dance and one definitely worth considering in the event that you might want to zero in on feeling glad and lively and reestablishing your delight for living yet favor something that offers somewhat more effect than the Oriental style of Dance for recuperating.

There are additionally mending water moves or hydrotherapy that are regularly utilized in assisting individuals with explicit wounds. These meetings are low effect however there is some level of obstruction offered through the water for extraordinary outcomes. You should make certain anyway that in the event that you are thinking about such a dance you have a certified teacher and if conceivable one on one consideration.

For some basic afflictions, there is a decent possibility that some type of dance exists that could help you in recuperating from your sickness. Also, there are frequently classes offered for bunches around there. In the event that you are thinking about figuring out how to move to improve your personal satisfaction or simply your delight in life by and large, I for one expectation you dance.

Ice Dance for Those Who Love a Challenge

For the individuals who love to move yet might want to take a stab at something somewhat more testing, there is consistently ice dance. This is a type of figure skating that additionally joins a portion of the standards and moves of couples dancing in with the general mish-mash for a smidgen of an additional test and a couple of more limitations with regards to moves and artistic freedom than conventional figure skating permits.

Ice dance additionally requires music that has an authoritative beat or style of cadence, which offers a couple of a greater number of limitations than conventional figure skating. Ice dance should be possible for no particular reason and happiness or as a feature of an opposition. The opposition in this wild however to some degree new (to American crowds at any rate) is very furious among overwhelm skaters and world pioneers in the field similar as customary figure skating.

Ice dance is an excellent and liquid type of dance that many consider to be significantly more elegant than either conventional formal dancing or customary figure skating. The specialized abilities just as the strength of each accomplice in this type of dance are very requesting and to become or stay serious in this style of dance one should continually attempt to home and improve one's abilities.

On the off chance that you have never had the chance to watch ice dance whether on TV or live, I recommend you accept the following accessible open door to do as such. Ice dance is an incredible method to go through the evening. It's a success with the young ladies in the event that you end up being a person. On the off chance that you end up being a father of little girls it will make you a legend in their eyes just as giving them other committed and persevering people to look to as saints also.

Regardless of whether you are too excited by the plunges, whirls, lifts, and flips you can't deny the devotion to art and game that these skaters should suffer to stay on top of their games. I can consider not many better saints I would prefer to have for my kids than competitors who commit such a lot of time, energy, and exertion to their games.

Watching ice dance is a pleasant route for some to go through an evening at home. Nonetheless, watching ice dance live is considerably more charming to numerous fans and onlookers. There is an energy and unity with the group that basically can't be handed-off through the TV screen. Being one of the observers at a live ice moving rivalry is nearly as energizing for me as being at a live game, for example, a football match-up or race.

There is an electric energy that accompanies being a piece of the horde of onlookers that is difficult to coordinate on screen or through some other medium. There is an immense contrast in hearing the thunder of a group or loud commendation through your TV and hearing everything around you as you sit in the center. It's a genuinely astounding and lowering experience.

Ice dance is a profoundly cutthroat game. On the off chance that you have a kid that is intrigued or you are intrigued yourself be set up to contribute a lot of time and cash into any genuine cutthroat endeavors that you may have in your future. As you have presumably assembled this is a joined forces rivalry. You should have an accomplice to really contend. This, for some is an additional wellspring of time and exertion. Not all accomplices are quick hits with each other and the science isn't generally there. Plan to contribute a decent arrangement of time and exertion into tracking down a decent accomplice for your ice dance endeavors if this is a game you genuinely wish to seek after. In the event that you simply need to partake as an observer notwithstanding, there is no accomplice required and a lot of diversion to be had.

Irish Step Dancing

On the off chance that you are searching for something a little new and distinctive with regards to moving, have you considered Irish advance moving? I'm certain that large numbers of you have known about if not seen shows, for example, "Riverdance" and different shows that show this delightful and interesting type of dance. "Master of the Dance" is another illustration of extraordinary Irish advance dance however it carries a more present day bend to the crowd.

In the event that you haven't had the chance to encounter this dance sensation live you should create an open door to do as such. This style of dance resembles none you've likely at any point seen previously. It is excellent and simultaneously unfathomably hard to take the actions that are required and show so little exertion. The energy engaged with these exhibitions is downright astounding.

Youthful and old the same are being surprised with regards to such a dance. The music is motivating and fun just like the means and kicks that are finished without breaking a sweat by the entertainers. In the event that you are searching for an incredible method to get a decent oxygen consuming exercise, check whether there is a class around there. This is a high energy type of dance and that ought to be recollected anyway you will get an incredible lower body exercise notwithstanding the high-impact benefits. You will likewise consume a decent numerous calories all the while.

This is a style of dance that essentially looks fun. Regardless of whether you are watching or partaking the fervor and energy level is practically apparent. It is out and out astonishing to be in the crowd for one of these shows. It ought to be added that while not all Irish advance moving requires the ability and energy that is found in the significant creations, for example, the ones I've referenced above, there is as yet a decent level of energy in all types of Irish advance moving. This energy is the thing that makes this way of moving so engaging.

Little youngsters, adolescents, and ladies across America are finding for themselves what a brilliant type of dance Irish advance moving truly is. These classes are somewhat more testing than some different types of moving might be on the grounds that they require the means to be made in accordance with different understudies in the class. You depend on one another and should stay up with the music. It is a great test that additionally helps understudies of this style of dance figure out how to cooperate as well as creating and refining their own Irish advance dance abilities. There are solo moves yet for the most striking influence these moves ought to be done as a feature of a bigger gathering. It really is a shocking incredible sight.

Assuming you have an enthusiasm for music and energy, maybe Irish advance moving classes would be a decent blend for you and your wellness and dance needs. It is a delightful way of moving that isn't simply enjoyable to observe yet additionally amusing to perform. You will work with a bigger gathering and figure out how to cooperate for the best conceivable impact. Of the multitude of styles of dance that are delighted in around the present reality, this is quite possibly the most fascinating types of gathering dance I've at any point experienced. On the off chance that you need to be a piece of something a lot bigger than yourself, this is an incredible method to do exactly that.

Jazz as Dance

While few individuals comprehend the genuine starting points of Jazz as a music structure, less individuals actually comprehend the beginnings of jazz as a style of dance. Jazz is a lot of a bastard kid. More than that notwithstanding, jazz as music and dance appear to have numerous moms regardless of the way that they have no dad. By this I imply that there are numerous impacts to this bright type of music and dance however nobody impact is outstanding enough in the new creation to be considered the 'father' or 'mother' besides of jazz.

Despite the fact that jazz has many guessed origin it truly just has one genuine home and that home would be New Orleans. Similar as the music this city is well known for, New Orleans is a city without a dad as well. New Orleans was a blend in the most genuine feeling of the word before we had any genuine piece of information what it intended to be a mixture. From the impacts of the French, Spanish, German, English, and obviously the number of inhabitants in previous slaves and dark free people, New Orleans was the ideal spot for this mixed constantly style of music and dance to call home.

It is no big surprise that jazz dance arose as the consequence of jazz music. There are basically no sufficient dance ventures for the magnificent music we have come to know over the course of the years as jazz. Therefore something new and a smidgen off the fundamental way was required to keep time and speed with the new music that was arising.

As a style of dance, jazz was substantially more 'baldfaced' than moves in the past had been and in certain circles viewed as independently uncalled-for. Respectable company surely had no interest in this specific type of dance. The uplifting news for the individuals who delighted in this style of dance is that there were a lot of spots where jazz, as a type of dance and music, was promptly embraced. You needed to go off in an unexpected direction somewhat to discover it however for some, it was certainly worth the exertion.

Jazz music and dance was well known for a long time and afterward appeared to go underground besides in urban areas like Memphis, New Orleans, Kansas City, and St. Louis where it was an instilled part of the set of experiences and culture. We have seen a reappearance of this previously well-known style of music and dance as of late anyway for certain striking performers bringing back the swing and 'huge band' sound that went connected at the hip with jazz as both a music structure and a style of dance.

You ought to see nonetheless, that with regards to jazz dance, similar as the music, there are no authoritative standards that you should continue with the end goal for it to be jazz. There are no unbending dance steps that should be clung to for the 'jazz' impact. Jazz dance is regularly befuddled as 'tap dance' since tap music was frequently set to jazz music. It is significant anyway to understand that jazz isn't restricted to tap dance and that different styles of dance fall under the fairly enormous umbrella of 'jazz dance'.

A portion of the more normal jazz moves include: Black Bottom, Boogie Woogie, the Cakewalk, the Charleston, the Jitterbug, the Lindy Hop, and swing moving. Every one of these styles of dance is by all accounts making a fairly amazing rebound in prominence throughout the most recent twenty years and are intriguing to watch, just as in which to take part should you at any point have the chance.

In the event that you have considered jazz dance exercises for you or your kids, I trust you will choose to enjoy. Not exclusively is the music for this kind of dance astounding and inspiring yet in addition the style of dance all by itself is very fun and pleasant. There are not very many styles of dance that can contend with regards to permitting creative liberty, accepting the way things are, and just moving for the sheer delight of moving. As a fine art and as a type of amusement jazz music and dance are tops in my book.

Figure out How to Dance

In the event that there is one thing in life that is certain it is this. Nobody is conceived realizing how to move. We as a whole have an inward ability to stay on beat and honestly some have it and some basically don't. The facts demonstrate that not every person is intended to move seriously and some won't ever refine their abilities enough to advance out of the mosh pit. Nonetheless, there are the individuals who have that internal feeling of equilibrium and musicality. With appropriate guidance and the correct motivation these individuals can possibly become remarkable artists.

Figuring out how to move is an interaction that turns out diversely for various individuals. Some learn best by one on one guidance. Others figure out how to adapt just by watching others dance. Some require a tad of rivalry to appropriately inspire themselves to stretch their boundaries and truly give moving their everything. Fortunately there are dance exercises and classes that are fitting for all extraordinary adapting needs with regards to move.

That being said, to move on a serious level almost certainly, you should consolidate a smidgen of all various techniques for educating and learning for the most ideal outcomes. There isn't anything amiss with watching others dance and taking in and getting motivation from the moves they make. You can likewise find defects, shortcomings, and errors by watching others move and gain from those also.

That being said, you won't ever gain as much from just watching different artists or guidelines on a video tape as you will in a study hall or one on one climate. Dance is liquid and there are sure details to the means yet there are different things included that mark the distinction between an artist with some level of specialized abilities and a genuinely incredible artist. A few things must be pushed and goaded from inside you and just a certified educator can truly achieve that.

The thing is most, who need to be artists, ought not make due with basically figuring out how to move. They need to figure out how to feel the music and utilize the music and their bodies to recount a story. That is what is the issue here. Not the execution of even muddled developments. Dance ought to be a passionate outlet more than all else. This is the manner in which dance has been since forever. It is just somewhat recently or with the goal that we have transformed dance into a game instead of a work of art and it has lost a portion of its intensity accordingly. The individuals who genuinely comprehend that genuine dance is conveying a message as opposed to conveying developments anyway are the victories that can't be coordinated.

On the off chance that you wish to figure out how to move, you need to painstakingly think about your explanations behind doing as such prior to settling on your technique for learning. I firmly suggest a tad bit of the multitude of various strategies. One thing to remember in any case, is that in the event that you gain from more than one educator you will be reprimanded for expecting to forget negative routines. It's a self image thing I accept. Most teachers incline toward rank amateurs with the goal that they don't need to 'unschool' any negative routines. Else, you ought to pick the teacher that you feel won't just show you how to move yet additionally urge you to move to the fullest of your latent capacity. Those are somewhat more hard to get.

Figure out How to Line Dance

There is a way of moving that is filling in prevalence significantly. While you are undeniably bound to see a line moving challenge at Gilley's than on ESPN or some other game organization, it doesn't make it any less legitimate as a dance or even as technique for bringing wellness back into the regular.

Line moving has been related basically with down home music for quite a while—best gauges say since the 170's. The uplifting news with line moving is that there aren't an excessive number of rules other than continue to attempt and don't spill your brew if there's anything you can do about it. Something else on the off chance that you will get stepped on for going the correct way or being stepped on by those going the incorrect way, it's an extraordinary method to go through an evening.

Line moving is extraordinary for some chuckles and loads of fun. It is in any case, significantly more fun in the event that you go in a gathering as opposed to going it single-handedly. This is one type of dance that you really should attempt before you can choose whether or not you will like it. I can sincerely say that watching others take part isn't close to as fun as being directly in the center of all and watching them take an interest.

The uplifting news for the individuals who aren't enlightened regarding the most recent advances, winds, turns, and moves, is that most other line artists started their excursion elsewhere too and are fairly understanding and regularly willing to instruct the individuals who are less proficient. Obviously in the event that they are in any way similar to me, they are so charmed to discover somebody less learned that they are practically overjoyed at the possibility of sharing their insight.

Far better for the absolute amateur is that most clubs offer exercises before things got truly jumping. Truth be told, the vast majority of these clubs will offer these exercises for no additional charge in order to sell you a pleasant cold a couple before prime selling time kicks in. You can likewise discover nearby gatherings that regularly offer line moving classes in a liquor free climate for the individuals who think about this as a significant thought and for a portion of the more youthful group that may discover line moving to be of interest.

Line moving is a style of dance that can be delighted in by individuals, all things considered, and wellness levels. This is one thing that makes it so broadly engaging. You can discover line moves at region fairs, nearby celebrations, and even church wagers every so often. Line moving is rapidly turning into a 'heartland' kind of amusement that is delighted in even by the individuals who aren't customarily down home music fans.

In all honesty women, line moving is likewise a fantastic method to convince your individual to hit the dance floor with you. Trust me when he sees you on the line with every one of those different folks he's most probable going to need to venture up and have a special interest. Obviously, it's additionally an extraordinary route for couples to have some good times together even in the center of a group. Line moving is incredible fun practically any way you take a gander at it. On the off chance that you are new to the idea of line moving there is no better time than right now to take off and get familiar. You could actually track down an extraordinary new interest that likewise ends up consuming a couple of calories simultaneously.

Figuring out how to Dance at Home

There are numerous manners by which an individual can figure out how to move on the off chance that the person in question is of the psyche to do as such. The issue is that numerous individuals avoid figuring out how to move, in spite of an earnest longing to do precisely that out of dread of being found in the learning interaction. This is a particularly tragic motivation to try not to bring the delight of dance into your life and one that can be so effectively stayed away from on the off chance that you will put forth the attempts that would be required.

Above all else, you can figure out how to move inside the solace of your own personal home. You needn't bother with a ballroom or studio with mirrors to figure out how to move despite the fact that they are useful to the interaction. Actually it is very conceivable to figure out how to move at home without getting an educator.

There are numerous DVDs and instructional tapes and recordings available that can show the nuts and bolts of various styles of dance. In the event that you don't know what sort of dance you are generally intrigued by, is anything but a horrendous plan to start by requesting a few DVDs to discover what explicit kind of dance intrigues you most. The truly slick thing about doing this is that you can being the learning cycle in your own personal home with the shades drawn and nobody will at any point should be any more astute.

Obviously in the event that you will learn at home you should hint your companion or accomplice in and check whether the person in question might want to go along with you on the way to finding the delights of dance as a type of diversion just as a methods for bringing an additional degree of active work into your life. The truly uplifting news is that such an active work will not feel like exercise and on the off chance that you do your best with your accomplice it could possibly prompt different types of active work. Remember that numerous individuals discover dance to be a heartfelt antecedent to other heartfelt pursuits.

Moving in an opposite direction from the sentiment office you can even track down an incredible and sporadically savage crowd in your youngsters. They likewise make extraordinary practice accomplices and guinea pigs and on the off chance that you control the remittance, you may even figure out how to crush out a commendation or two to help your conceivably injured personality through the occasion. Children are incredible fun however with regards to moving and (more youthful children at any rate) are quite often able to kick back and enjoy a chuckle at mother or fathers cost. On the off chance that you need to make a truly fun evening of things, challenge your children to a 'dance off' you could actually be shock at who is the last one standing.

Figuring out how to move at home can be a compensating experience in the event that you apply the things you learn. In addition to the fact that you get the advantage of another diversion you figure out how to do as such without the vulnerability and weakness that is frequently a typical piece of exercises. Having a group of people can be something startling, in any case, whenever you've breezed through the kid assessment you ought to be prepared for the most savage crowd any dance studio can give. You ought to likewise remember that different understudies in the class (should you at any point conclude you are prepared to take a real class) are presumably similarly as anxious about their degree of ability as you might be.

Figuring out how to Love to Dance

Of the relative multitude of endowments you can give your kids on the planet training them to very much want to move is one of the best. Moving is an extraordinary method to get your kids dynamic, keep them solid, and in numerous occurrences, keep them cheerful. Since the beginning dance has been supposed to be an overt gesture of happiness. I would imagine that happiness and an approach to communicate it is a superb heritage to leave our kids.

Indeed, even Shakespeare comprehended the significance of dance and the delight that dance was intended to be the outflow of.

"To sing them as well: when you do move, I wish you

A wave o' the ocean, that you may at any point do"

- The Winter's Tale

In these words, this was a wish of extraordinary significance and intended to be favorable luck to the one that was the object of the loving wish. It appears to be that incidentally nonetheless, awfully many have failed to remember the incredible blessing that moving truly is for the brain, the body, and the spirit of man and lady the same.

Encouraging your kids to very much want to move will give them the establishment for a solid way of life that is lower in pressure than large numbers of their companions and colleagues en route will at any point know. It will ingrain in them the worth of order and commitment alongside the sheer delight of just moving to the music. Not every person is intended to move on a cutthroat level yet I can't in any way, shape or form accept that we were planned as we were and not intended to move.

Figuring out how to very much want to move is likewise the best blessing you can give yourself. Similar as your kids you need to bring actual wellness into your life. You need to reaffirm the significance of control in your life. The greater part of us need to assuage a portion of the pressure that is in our lives and we as a whole need to set aside somewhat more effort for ourselves and focus on recuperating and recharging our own spirits instead of expenditure the entirety of our accessible energy sustaining and rejuvenating others.

We need to figure out how to very much want to move as a source for repressed feeling just as the chance to work out those things that drive us from the inside. We need dance as a strategy for fighting with ourselves and as a method of communicating our own delights and wins. Dance is a fantastic methods for these things thus significantly more.

There is nothing of the sort as being excessively sound. Dance can help lower pulse, increment dissemination, improve muscle tone, and essentially cause you to feel more vivacious and invigorated. There are not many things that can contend with the fortification of moving. Figuring out how to very much want to move gives you the ideal chance to improve your general wellbeing and wellness level without feeling like you have accomplished something incorrectly all the while. This is no lose circumstance for the individuals who have nothing to lose other than a couple of pounds that have waited unreasonably long.

Presently is the ideal time for you to start the way toward figuring out how to very much want to move. Whenever you've figured out how to very much want to move you need to impart that affection and enthusiasm to those you love. This would be your loved ones. Dance together, play together, and live more, more joyful coexistences.

Music About Dance

While we as a whole realize that Jazz is as much a style of music as it is a style of dance, numerous individuals may not understand the significance that dance has played in music. There are numerous melodies out there that notice the significance of moving but we as a general public appear to have failed to remember the significance or restricted that significance to a specific age bunch. When we age it appears to be that we fail to remember how to move as well as the inborn significance of moving too.

"I Hope You Dance" is just one of numerous melodies that relate the significant job that moving plays in taking care of the human spirit. In the event that one thing in life is significant for all, that one thing is dance at whatever point the chance emerges. No one can tell whenever you will run out of freedoms to move or find that you've wasted so many of them away. Accept them surprisingly your life will be loaded up with a lot more noteworthy delight than you may at any point figure it out. Regardless of numerous different tunes out there that may pass on the message, there are not very many that say it more succinctly than this specific tune. "At the point when you get the decision to pass on it or dance, I trust you'll move".

Garth Brooks is another artist that had a phenomenal discourse on dance. His melody "The Dance" accounts not really the significance of moving but rather of taking an interest. Given the decision, numerous who have lost their lives in some dangerous undertaking would without a doubt tell those left behind that they would not have exchanged the dance for one more breath. The verses to this melody are to some degree frequenting "I might have missed the agony however I'd have needed to miss the dance".

In all honesty all great melodies that notice dance don't turn out to be blue grass tunes. These genuinely end up being, as I would see it, the most impactful. Other extraordinary tunes about dance incorporate the melody "We should Dance" by David Bowie. The verses to this tune incorporate the refrain "How about we dance for dread around evening time is all". The reality of the situation is that you never know and moving is an incredible method to praise living.

Music and dance for quite a long time have gone inseparably and will keep on doing so long after we've left this world. In any event that would be the expectation. I would prefer not to perceive what a world without dance would resemble. It would resemble having kids without chuckling and that would be a pitiful world wherein to live. On the off chance that you need to keep your youngsters moving, you should instruct them to move. Instruct them that it is alright to move and be senseless around the house. That it is OK to move their way through their errands (hello on the off chance that it makes them grin while making a garbage run I say pull out all the stops!). Instruct them that moving is an extraordinary method to communicate delight and that chuckling is the best thing to follow their dance.

Local Americans have a long and honorable legacy with regards to move. They let their fantasies thump out the heartbeat of Mother Earth and moved in friendship with nature. They moved for happiness and distress, war, harmony, and recognition. I can think about no better guide to follow with regards to move.

Choosing the Proper Dance Shoes

In the event that you've at any point been to a wedding or prom in awkward shoes you know the significance of this interaction. You totally should choose agreeable shoes in the event that you intend to move for a significant stretch of time. Having those perfect thump me dead heels is fine and dandy for the image part of your evening however when you're moving you will need to be wearing shoes that you can really move around in without needing to cry. Other than who truly needs to chance a mascara stream for the after prom party?

On the off chance that you need to be certain whether your prom shoes will be agreeable for the large dance occasion take a stab at moving around the house in them at throughout the hours of the day and night. Ensure that there is no squeezing, scouring, or rankling therefore or your will spend by far most of your prom late evening remaining uninvolved as opposed to hitting the dance floor with your date. Similar remains constant for weddings. Pictures are just fine, so is making that shocking passage. Simultaneously there isn't anything very like being the last one standing with regards to the dance floor.

I'm a firm adherent to adorable shoes. I'm additionally a firm adherent to having agreeable feet. Suggestions for impact point tallness are that 2 inches are really the awesome offering curve help and foot wellbeing notwithstanding solace. Indeed, this implies that this stature is really suggested over wearing pads. You'll likewise need to ensure there is a lot of room in the toe territory so your foot has a little breathing space without permitting space to rub and possibly rankle. At the end of the day a cozy (yet not tight) fit is desirable over shoes that fit freely. You ought to have your shoes for the large occasion appropriately estimated.

On the off chance that you just can't leave behind the beautiful 4 inch stilettos you found marked down as the ideal ally for your prom or wedding dress, at that point you ought to at any rate consider a back up pair of shoes that will be considerably more agreeable once the passageway has been make, the photos have been taken, and you lose all feeling of feeling in your feet. It is very hard to make convoluted dance step when the voice in your mind is shouting "Ouch! Ouch!" with each and every progression you make. Your shoes will really influence pretty much every once of satisfaction you experience for the evening there is no explanation you should wear awkward shoes and be hopeless for an evening that should be enjoyable.

You should look at dance stores in an around your old neighborhood and see what they have to bring to the table. They make shoes that are above all else intended to be moved in. They additionally make some exceptionally cheeky shoes that are totally fitting for formals and would be very reasonable to wear to a wedding or prom. You can discover these shoes on the web however I advise against this as you can't get them appropriately fitted on the web and it doesn't make any difference how incredible they are planned if the shoes don't fit as expected, they are very liable to hurt your feet. Interestingly, you set aside the effort to discover shoes that you feel will be agreeable for moving without forfeiting the look you are endeavoring to assemble.

So You Think You can Dance

On the off chance that you are a fanatic of unscripted tv chances are that you have known about the hit show on Fox by the name of "So You Think You can Dance". In the event that you are a fanatic of "American Idol" this show could very well additionally be of enticement for you. It is similar as the uncontrollably well known Fox hit, American Idol just the attention is on dance as opposed to vocal abilities.

Similar as American Idol, So You Think You can Dance has a tryout cycle by which the wheat is isolated from the refuse as it were. The initial two scenes of the period are basically cuts from the tryout interaction showing a portion of the hits and misses that have been experienced all through the way toward trimming down the numbers. It should come as no colossal shock that Simon from American Idol is additionally one of the makers for this show which is well known by its own doing however not arriving at anyplace close to the wild achievement that American Idol has encountered.

This show will utilize artists with a wide scope of foundation. From road entertainers to those that have recently held titles for their moving abilities, they start on an even and level battleground and are dispensed with as the opposition escalates and swarm assumptions rise. The prize for winning on this arrangement is $100,000 cash, a moving part in the Las Vegas show of Celine Dion and their very own Hybrid SUV (I do praise the endeavors of the makers to settle on greener decisions in this matter incidentally).

The show is quite fascinating on a level that American Idol doesn't figure out how to catch. For one, it includes the matching up of ability that hasn't cooperated already with the end goal of dance while going up against each other. Furthermore, they most minimal scoring couple is permitted the chance for one part to vindicate oneself by performing solo for the appointed authorities. Clearly this makes for some intriguing circumstances en route. One more intriguing reality about this show is that it tosses the contenders into types of dance that they are not liable to be acquainted with against different entertainers who might just be comfortable and OK with the style of dance being referred to.

All things considered, with regards to move, the network show So You Think You can Dance is doing an incredible arrangement to teach its watchers about different styles of dance that they may have never in any case experienced. In the event that you have for a long while been itching to gain proficiency with somewhat more about the numerous styles of dance and to consider others to be they get acquainted with everything somewhat, at that point this is unquestionably a show you will not have any desire to miss.

I ought to likewise accept this open door to bring up that shows, for example, Dancing with the Stars on ABC additionally gives a fantastic setting to instruction and diversion with regards to move. In this arrangement VIPs are really combined with proficient partner dancers and put through a dance hall 'training camp' of sorts to become familiar with the artistic work of traditional dancing at that point put through a lot with judges and citizens the same. In truth, any openness to the magnificent craft of dance is something beneficial for some, who are conquering their assumptions about dance.

The Incredible Importance of Dance

Since the commencement of the world, dance has assumed an essential part in probably the most significant and life changing festivals and functions that have existed. Fights have been battled and won quickly following weapons moves, Kingdoms have been one and lost and celebrated with moves. Lords and Monarchs have been delegated then celebrated with moves, and relationships have been culminated with moves of another sort.

Dance has consistently been at the focal point of significant occasions until ongoing history when doubtlessly dance and the significance of dance to resolve has been lost some place all the while. Dance these days is by all accounts restricted to specific individuals in specific conditions or just to the individuals who take part in the craft of dance for the diversion of others as opposed to the straightforward delight of moving for moving.

Dance is a unique little something that ought not be a reference in the diaries of the historical backdrop of the world. At the point when humanity looses the capacity to move for bliss, there truly is no justification the race of humankind to forge ahead. The capacity to move, as an overt gesture of feeling is one of those uncommon things that isolates a man from a monster.

In spite of the fact that the significance of dance appears to have been lost somewhat recently or something like that, we are seeing a resurrection of sorts for the love of dance lastly starting to see a portion of the more significant issues that dance addresses. It is undeniably more than something intended to engage onlookers. It ought to likewise engage those that are doing the moving.

Notwithstanding the amusement part of dance, which ought not be lessened, dance is additionally an actual work. We experience a daily reality such that the normal life expectancy of our youngsters, is more limited than the life expectancy of the individuals who are as of now grown-ups. The essential justification this is an absence of actual wellness and an excess of weight. We need to show others how its done and show our kids that it is critical to do easily overlooked details that get us off our seats and moving around. Dance is an incredible method to do precisely that.

Past this notwithstanding, dance has other wellness benefits. By expanding your muscle tone and your blood stream by moving you are giving your heart a 'battery help' as it were. Doing this consistently will lead your heart to be a lot better heart than if you somehow happened to lead a stationary way of life. Dance additionally eases pressure and deliveries endorphins if your burning some calories as it were. This causes you to feel glad and cases and diminishes cases of sorrow.

Another incredible advantage of dance to the individuals who care is the way that it expands muscle tone and gives your body a more drawn out and more slender investigate time and with reliable, restrained preparing. Some have likewise seen a restored feeling of beauty and continually expanding self-assurance.

Obviously, if these reasons aren't sufficient to persuade you regarding the significant job that dance can play in your life just as in the public eye then maybe you ought to simply get out there and dance. Give it a shot, perceive how much fun it is to move for reasons unknown other than to move and afterward attempt to clarify why we as a general public don't have to take part in such exercises somewhat more regularly.

The Wedding Dance

All throughout the planet couples commend their associations with a wedding dance or something to that affect. Most religions, except for the individuals who actually dislike moving, have a type of wedding dance that is a piece of this cheerful occasion or the festival of this occasion. This is considerably more than a basic dance. The dance will start your life as a couple. Hence alone, numerous couples invest a lot of energy and exertion picking the ideal melody to represent their affection for each. When concluded, this is the tune that will be played for their wedding dance.

Your wedding dance is one of only a handful few recollections of your wedding that you will have until the end of time. The majority of your big day will pass by in such a haze of countenances that there will be few seconds that stand apart over the rest. Your wedding dance in any case, is the one time during your wedding gathering that you and your life partner are really alone inside the group. Everyone's eyes might be on you both however this is your second together and nobody else in the room should matter right now. This is the explanation that a great many people will recollect their wedding dance long after they've failed to remember different insights regarding their wedding.

A few couples really take wedding dance exercises to ensure that nothing turns out badly during their wedding dance. Numerous teachers regularly propose that you utilize the shoes you will be wearing for your wedding just as a skirt that is basically the same as your wedding dress to really get a legitimate feel for how you will move on your big day. It is stunning the amount of a distinction the tallness of your shoes and the length of your skirt or train can make with regards to moving.

These classes are vital for couples that genuinely need to have the fantasy wedding experience however not really viable for couples that are now working toward the finish of their spending requirements.

Couples dance exercises will regularly do the trick for wedding dance exercises and as a rule are considerably less costly on the off chance that you can take them at a neighborhood public venue instead of taking private exercises. Gathering exercises are quite often more efficient and can be an extraordinary route for you and your future companion to figure out how to move together on schedule for your enormous evening and your wedding dance.

In the event that financial plans will not take into consideration this guilty pleasure to make your wedding dance somewhat simpler to deal with you can generally select to buy an instructional video or DVD. It would be incredible enjoyable to rehearse your wedding dance together before the large evening and it is an extraordinary method to have a great time all together even after the huge evening. You can discover recordings and DVDs that show all way of dance steps that you may discover engaging.

Else you can continually make things up along the way. Pick a tune you love, a dance you like and have a great time without stressing over getting it awesome. You are starting your new coexistence as a team and who actually needs the pressing factor of moving great, isn't that so? It is likewise your day and that is one thing that excessively couple of ladies truly acknowledge when becoming involved with the pressing factor of making the ideal wedding inside a restricted financial plan.

The thing to recollect when arranging your wedding and your wedding dance is that you and your life partner to be are the main individuals simultaneously. Try not to permit yourself to feel constrained into something that you don't need to mollify others. Make your big day and your wedding dance totally your own on the off chance that you are not inspired by or OK with taking exercises from another person. You and your accomplice will be happy that you made the right decision for you no matter what.

Why Dance?

With regards to move there are numerous reasons that various individuals in various societies traversing the globe decide to move. This article will investigate a portion of the numerous reasons that individuals dance all throughout the planet and maybe give new motivators to you to move your way during your time also.

Moving for Religion

Numerous religions all throughout the planet and since forever have utilized dance in recognition of their divinities, in festival of the seasons, and essentially as an overt gesture of delight. Christianity has blended feelings with regards to move. A few religions feel that all way of social dance can prompt prohibited activities or musings and will in general disapprove of dance overall subsequently while other Christian religions accept that there is a period, spot, and reason for moving. Some have even joined moving into their strict functions (weddings as one model). Most will concur that dance involves individual conviction inside the Christian religion in view of the warmed discussions that can emerge on the subject.

The Hindu religion dance is a fundamental type of adoring the different parts of the Divine. This type of dance is regularly erroneously alluded to as Classical Indian Dance however truly it is a type of love. There are various moves for the various gods as each god has an alternate inclination.

Indeed, even the religion of Islam has its own form of moving for love. The individuals who practice this type of dance for love are regularly alluded to as Whirling Dervishes.

The Weapon Dance

This is a type of dance that has a long history tracing all the way back to Spartan fighters getting ready for the fight to come. This style of dance has been utilized from the beginning of time and all throughout the planet by numerous countries and societies as readiness, preparing, and raising spirit for up and coming fight. In spite of the fact that not, at this point broadly rehearsed, and surely not as a forerunner to fight, the set of experiences and service of the Weapon Dance isn't to be neglected and still rehearsed in stately occasions today to respect the manner in which things have been done previously.

Local American Tribal Dances

It is additionally significant that what has gotten usually alluded to as war moves by Native American clans are perhaps exactly the same weapons moves that have a long and honorable history all throughout the planet. Singular clans had their own moves that were utilized when getting ready to fight with different clans, planning for a major chase, or planning to guard themselves against steady attack and migration.

War, or inescapable fight was not by any means the only explanation that Native American clans moved notwithstanding. Dance held a significant job in the venerating of different divine beings just as ancestral services or individual articulations of petition, melancholy, happiness, or basically of accepting nature and become one with their general surroundings. Dance is fundamental for Native American legacy and culture. For Native American dance, the beat of the drum is a fundamental part. The drumbeat drives the speed and the power of the dance.

Serious Dance

All throughout the planet there are those that dance seriously in all types of dance. From sporting types of moving to otherworldly types of moving the rivalries are savage and the contenders regularly devote their lives and by far most of their available energy to sharpening and culminating their specific types of dance. In aggressive dance there are judges who judge imaginative articulation, specialized abilities, ensembles, and the consistency or execution of developments. The individuals who dance seriously should be focused on their art to stay cutthroat.

Obviously a few group dance essentially on the grounds that they need to and there is positively nothing amiss with that. There is actually no terrible motivation to move except if you are being compelled to do as such without wanting to. In any case with regards to move, the best motivation to move is on the grounds that the music leaves you no other alternative except for to move.

Why Not Dance?

There are some strict restrictions with regards to move other than strict reasons why for heaven's sake would anybody not have any desire to encounter the psyche and body reestablishing energy that outcomes from moving? Honestly, not all moving includes the wearing of pink tutus and numerous types of dance are very manly in nature so safeguarding manliness can't in any capacity be a satisfactory pardon for not moving.

With regards to move there are many intriguing and stunning styles of dance that range the globe. From the weapon moves of old (which are an ideal showcase of virility and manliness however not broadly rehearsed today other than in stylized dance) to the elegance and magnificence of artful dance or partner dancing there is practically sure to be some type of dance that should engage nearly anybody in the world.

Local Americans had a great disposition and beliefs with regards to moving. They moved for practically any explanation and let the beat of the drum fill in as their directing soul. Local Americans moved for love, for downpour, for euphoria, for anguish, and to get ready for war. Their moves were sincere and as much a piece of their individual qualities as it was their ancestral personalities. Moving was a fundamental piece of their way of life and legacy is as yet given today however to a lot more modest degree.

While a few religions debilitate dance, others embrace dance as a type of love and obligation to their gods. Some empower dance as an outflow of applause. Others dance for the delight of the endowments and abundance of their divine beings or in accommodation to their divine beings. Notwithstanding the reality stays that dance assumes an imperative part in a significant number of the world's religions. In the event that you are a devotee, I can consider not many preferable motivations to move over to communicate your convictions in an actual structure.

A few group dance just on the grounds that they like music and appreciate watching others dance. There are a wide range of fun moving styles that can be drilled alone, as a couple, or as a piece of a lot bigger gathering. In the United States line moving and square moving are brilliant approaches to move as a component of a bigger gathering just as numerous sorts of serious moving and as a feature of an artful dance organization or other kind of aggressive or expert dance organization. Couples moving somewhat incorporates square moving however different types of dance, for example, formal dancing also. Singles moving is basically saved to serious moving and regularly requires long periods of training to consummate. A few group dedicate their lives to such a moving and still never figure out how to positively influence the serious moving circuit.

Moving for wellness is another wave that is by all accounts surprising the world. There are numerous ways that this should be possible and it is very successful among the individuals who might some way or another not exercise at all just as the individuals who basically love to move. It is escaping your seat and moving around to the music. Track down a decent driving beat, close the shades, and dance until you can no longer breath. It's an incredible method to get that truly necessary exercise while having some good times and not in any event, understanding that you are (wheeze) working out. Psyche over issue is something incredible. Assuming it doesn't feel like exercise, there is no justification your body, psyche, or soul to dissent, isn't that so?

Moving is turning out to be to some degree a curiosity sport around the USA and all throughout the planet. Unscripted tv shows, for example, "Hitting the dance floor with Stars" and motion pictures, for example, the one with Richard Gere—Shall We Dance have made couples dancing mainstream and appealing to the normal individual who might have never thought to be this type of dance. With such countless great explanations behind an individual to move why in the world wouldn't you need to move?

Don't miss out!

Visit the website below and you can sign up to receive emails whenever Mary Stephens publishes a new book. There's no charge and no obligation.

https://books2read.com/r/B-A-MESO-VVROB

BOOKS 2 READ

Connecting independent readers to independent writers.

Also by Mary Stephens

Beauty Books: Are They Worth Your Money?
A Quick and Easy Guide on Dance